SWITCHING TO A VEGAN LIFESTYLE

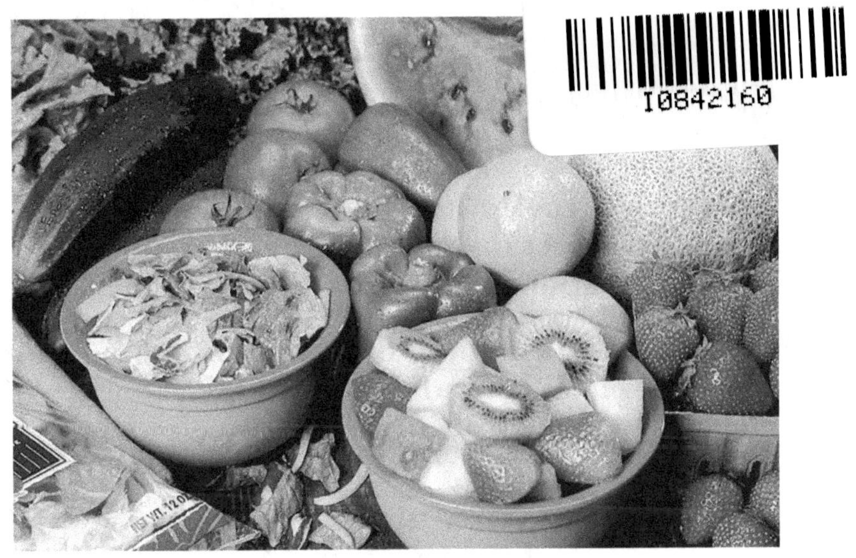

M. A. HILL

DISCLAIMER

Neither the author's nor the publisher assumes any responsibilities for errors, omission or contrary interpretation of the subject matter herein.

This book is for entertainment. The views expressed are those of the author alone and should not be taken as expert instruction or commands. The reader is responsible for his or her own actions.

This book is dedicated to those committed to a more healthy and conscious life.

Author

"If slaughterhouses had glass walls, everyone would be a vegetarian."

Paul McCartney

Table of Contents

INTRODUCTION

The vegan lifestyle is a healthy way of living. Eating habits of vegan people are slightly different from vegetarians who abstain from consuming meat products, while vegans not only avoid eating animal flesh, they also refrain from eating food stuffs derived from animals, such as eggs, dairy products, and honey. Leading a vegan lifestyle also means that people don't use cosmetics tested on animals.

Significant health benefits are derived from a plant-based diet that is naturally low in cholesterol and fat, but high in fiber. People following the vegan lifestyle find that the risk of certain chronic diseases is minimized. Consuming a meat-free diet significantly increases quality of life and ensures a greater life span.

People following a vegan diet are normally free from all irritating allergens that may result in food allergies, asthma, and ADHD. This diet also supports aesthetically pleasing healthy hair, lowers body weight, and builds clearer, taut, and glowing skin. Therefore, people are gradually converting to a vegan life style for reasons even beyond health.

They also envision this way of living as precluding cruelty. Vegans believe that by excluding animal products from their diet, more plant food will be grown for human consumption, creating a better environment for all.

In this manner, the individual contributes to creating a green and clean environment, while also helping eliminate the useless slaughter of animals for food.

Scientists believe that the menace of Global warming, shortage of water, and deforestation are linked to the livestock industry, so promoting the vegan lifestyle is an environmentally friendly and socially ethical thing to do. It is estimated that animal excrement accounts for 18% of greenhouse gas emissions.

The benefits of a vegan diet become all the more pronounced when people start cooking their own meals, as vegan meals are served in a limited number of restaurants. People also become more aware of nutrition and begin to understand the positive effects of the diet high in plant fiber that lays the foundation of a healthier lifestyle.

Following the vegan lifestyle is an ideal way of gifting family a nutritious diet plan that can lead to significant health benefits. It is also budget-friendly, as plant food is less expensive than dairy products and meat.

Healthwise, vegan living appears to be gaining in popularity, and environmentally there is less risk of contaminating land or water, thereby allowing vegans to contribute, in a small way, towards preserving nature.

Discover effective ways of transitioning into a vegan lifestyle in this AMAZING GUIDE developed especially for you.

What are you waiting for?

LET'S GET STARTED!

CHAPTER 1

WHAT IS VEGANISM?

Veganism is a way of life for many. It is a lifestyle or dietary choice where a person abstains completely from all animal-based products, including meat, fish, eggs, cheese, milk, butter, cream, and honey.

Some individuals who adopt veganism will also go beyond dietary boundaries and ensure that their entire way of life is consistent with treating animals with kindness and respect, such as abstaining from purchasing leather or fur garments and bags, and not purchasing any products such as make-up, kitchenware, or furniture where animals have been used to make or test these products in any way.

Being vegan offers the opportunity to expand your culinary choices, but you don't need to if you prefer not to. A meat eater could still have his or her (faux) meat and 3 veggies every night without the guilt or immorality associated with an actual meat-based diet.

Most of the day-to-day ingredients we consumed as meat eaters have a veggie substitute, be it vitamins found in vegetables and nuts or faux cheeses and meats.

Milk on cereal, in coffee or tea, and in breakfast and cooking is easily replaced with the many non-dairy types that can be found at health stores such as rice, oat and soy milks. There are egg, meat and cheese substitutes to ensure that no traditional home-cooked meal needs to be missed.

Many who decide to convert to an exclusively plant-based vegan diet decide to keep their already-purchased leather, wool and silk garments until they are old and worn out.

Often, these people argue that this is because they feel that an animal had to die and suffer in the production of the product and therefore it should not have died in vain. Others decide that it's repulsive to wear dead animal products and cannot bear the sight of the product anymore.

Ultimately, the choice to wear out or throw out is up to each individual. Over time, however, most vegans will eventually rid themselves of all their ignorant or unconcerned purchases. They have comfort in knowing that they no longer support or condone these cruel and senseless industries.

Being vegan can be very challenging, especially when it comes to the attitudes of other non-vegan friends, family, and co-workers.

Unless you are blessed to be surrounded by enlightened vegans, you will more than likely be ridiculed, told that you will make yourself ill, that man was designed to eat animals, or that you're just plain weird. Some people you know may be in shock and won't understand your decision.

All new vegans will eventually find their own responses that they feel comfortable with and that work for them. But do try to avoid being adversarial, as this may offend others and damage the cause for veganism. It's best to adopt an engaging and positive approach to vegan advocacy wherever possible.

As a vegan, you will need to consume certain foods to ensure optimal health. It is essential to ensure that you get enough protein, calcium, iron, and vitamin B12 in your diet. It is best to gain these nutrients from food itself, however, there are also vitamin supplements available at most health stores.

Whatever your personal reasons for becoming a vegan, I'd like to assure you that you've made the right choice. Making the transition can appear daunting to some people but do not despair - you are not alone.

There are more like-minded and famous vegans than you might imagine, and their numbers grow as more people become aware of the benefits of being vegan.

CHAPTER 2

ADVANTAGES OF BEING A VEGAN

Regardless if you are looking to make a massive change or just a few small adjustments, vegan cooking can offer a great number of benefits, which helps many people pick up the habit.

Aside from the reality that a vegan lifestyle is much more green than eating tons of meat, it also has the huge benefit of being a much cheaper lifestyle.

Because the majority of the foods that are eaten in the vegan lifestyle can be grown at home, it provides a substantial savings that you would not otherwise be able to realize if you were relying on purchasing all your foods from a grocery store.

By omitting meats from your diet, you are not only doing your part to help the environment but with potential savings in the thousands of dollars possible each year, it can be a huge benefit to look towards a Vegan lifestyle.

Other concerns that are important is the ability to avoid chemically treated foods. Many vegans opt to grow their own produce, which provides the huge benefit of allowing you to use your own home-grown organic foods. This makes them much cheaper for you, which again can significantly decrease your average food expense.

It's a great idea to go vegan for many reasons.

Deeper compassion

A vegan's compassion extends to all living creatures. With increased compassion comes greater acceptance of all life and the appreciation that it adds value to our own, making us stronger.

Expanded palate

Vegans learn to enjoy a very wide range of vegetables, which leads to an expanded palate. Recipes abound for cooking every vegetable imaginable. When veggies are just a side dish, it's convenient to settle for a few of them to complement meat, such as potato salad, peas and carrots, or corn. Once veggies are the main dish, however, one starts to appreciate many more ingredients, enriching the dining experience.

Global impact

The vegan lifestyle is much more than food. It's about the environment, climate, sustainable development, efficient allocation of food sources, and animal welfare. Many of the themes associated with going green are linked to veganism.

When one chooses to be vegan, one participates and supports these themes. The impact of eating vegan is so powerful that if everyone did it constantly or even occasionally, many of these issues would resolve themselves.

Increased mobility

Nutritionists, dietitians, and health scientists are confirming the health benefits of a plant-based diet over a meat-based one. Lower blood pressure, reduced risk of heart disease and cancer, and longer life spans are possible outcomes with a vegan diet. Fewer health problems mean that one is more active and mobile and can enjoy life more fully.

Larger social network

The vegan community is large and growing. Vegans enjoy sharing their experiences and finding companions who understand the reasons for their eating habits. Meeting and connecting with new people is one of the fun social aspects of being vegan.

New knowledge

The vegan diet is focused on ingredients, health, and nutrition. To enjoy vegan food and stay healthy, one inevitably learns more about nutrition and the impact of ingredients on health.

Over time, by paying attention to what is consumed and the value of each ingredient, one becomes familiar with vitamins, minerals, protein, fiber, antioxidants, and phytonutrients, with which comes new knowledge and power.

Veganism is a lifestyle choice that today is accepted as normal by more and more people. Many people don't feel ready or willing to make the change, but if you have determined that veganism is for you, you may find it very worthwhile.

CHAPTER 3

WHAT DO VEGANS EAT?

While many people today are fully aware of the advantages of eating vegan, they are somehow hesitant to becoming vegan because of the food restrictions imposed by the vegan diet. This fear of restriction is probably what deters most the people.

They only think of what vegans can't eat, rather than valuing what vegans can eat. They only view the Vegan diet from one perspective without considering another point of view.

Vegans can eat a wide, interesting variety of foods. The list goes from vegetables down to eating pizza, chocolate chips cookies, and salads.

These dishes are suitable for vegans as long as they are made entirely from plant-based ingredients and definitely no animal ingredients. The only limitation for vegans is not eating any products made from animals, as they support the welfare of animals. Other than that, the vegan diet is as good and interesting as any diet.

So, what do vegans really eat?

This □uestion is perhaps the most common question people ask. This seems to be a common concern and it has almost become a joke among vegans that this □uestion is asked over and over again, and we have all heard it at one time or another.

Here is a list of foods that vegans eat. It is impossible to name all vegan foods, but in this chapter, I will name a few.

Tofu - this is made from soybeans. Tofu is naturally low in carbohydrates and fat and is a very rich source of protein. Tofu is very versatile and can be cooked in many ways. It can be used in snacks or meals and even be used in some desserts.

Vegetables - Preferably the yellow-orange and deep green ones. A great example of this is white and sweet potatoes. Be sure to eat fresh vegetables. Frozen vegetables are only second-best nutritionally.

Tempeh – this is also made from soybeans, specifically from fermented soybeans. Though this description may not sound too appetizing, the product is tasty and nutty. Tempeh is often served sliced and can be eaten as is.

Pastas - pasta are made from flour and water. There are also whole grain products such as spaghetti and macaroni made from whole wheat, spinach, artichokes, and corn.

Fruits - Apples are the best fruits, along with citrus fruits. Eat fruits during breakfast and be sure they are fresh.

Legumes - these are dry beans and peas. Excellent choices for this include garbanzos, black and red beans, and lentils.

Grains - Whole grains such as oats, brown rice, and whole wheat are the best examples of this. Eat as many as you can.

Nuts and Seeds - source of good fats and other good things.

Always bear in mind that these four foods: fruits, vegetables, nuts, and grains and legumes comprises the vegan diet. The vegan diet is not as restrictive as people assume it is. There is an endless list of vegan foods that provide plenty of nutrients and vitamins.

CHAPTER 4

VEGAN MYTHS AND TRUTHS

Once you've resolved to become vegan, the next step in your plan should be to arm yourself with veggie factoids. You can expect your friends, family, and coworkers to bombard you with □uestions about veganism and your new and improved lifestyle.

And chances are, some will be skeptical. I will provide you with a bit of myth-busting so you can give them the what's what when it comes to a vegan diet.

1: A vegan diet lacks sufficient protein, iron, and calcium.

Truth: A well-balanced vegan diet has more than enough nutrients. Beans, lentils, and soy are the protein standbys, although protein is also found in vegetables and starches.

And when it comes to calcium and iron, plant-based foods like nuts and seeds, tofu, beans, leafy greens and other foods sources are full of them in forms that are actually better absorbed by the body. As long as you consume enough calories by varying your vegan meals, your iron, calcium, and protein needs will be easily met.

2: Vegans only eat salad.

Truth: With vegan meals like grilled flank steak, Italian sausage and peppers, and even grilled mahi mahi out there without a trace of dairy, meat, pork, or fish, today's vegans should have no trouble finding something delicious and nutritious to eat.

More and more restaurants and online vegan delivery services are offering decadent and complex vegan meals that would please even the heartiest meat eaters.

3: Vegan food is hard to find and prepare.

Truth: Vegans have a wide variety of "normal" and delicious food choices easily available. In any typical American restaurant or supermarket, you can usually find an excellent selection of foods that are vegan friendly. And many ethnic restaurants such as Thai, Chinese, Vietnamese, Indian, and Ethiopian have plenty of vegan foods on the menu.

At home, your choices are unlimited. Like meat eaters, not all vegans eat the same way. While some stick to non-traditional foods like tofu and soy products, many vegans eat a lot of traditional dishes the vegan way. It's easy to take a non-vegan dish, such as cheese lasagna or bakery items and modify it by replacing the non-vegan ingredients with plant-based ones instead.

And these old favorites often end up tasting just like the original. Don't forget to take advantage of online vegan meals delivery services, which can take the guesswork out of the whole veganism process.

4: A vegan diet is expensive.

Truth: Vegetables and grains are less expensive than meat, period. Since plants grow in soil, they're ready to go as soon as they're ripe. That means less production cost.

To produce meat, you start with plants grown from the earth, pick them when they're ripe, feed them to an animal, fatten it up, kill the animal, and then it's ready to go. You could even start buying fresh, expensive-looking fruit you see in the specialty produce section instead of blowing all that cash on a pound of meat.

CHAPTER 5

THE DIFFERENCE BETWEEN A VEGAN AND A VEGETARIAN

Veganism is a way of living that seeks to exclude, as far as possible and practicable, all forms of exploitation of and cruelty to animals for food, clothing, and any other purpose.

This means that vegans don't eat cows, pigs, chicken, fish, or other such animals, as well as any broths, sauces, or gravies made from them. Beyond that, vegans also avoid eating all animal products, such as milk, butter, cheese, eggs, and honey.

Certain foods like Jell-O contain gelatin, a substance made from ground cow and horse hooves, and vegans avoid these as well, in addition to other animal products like glycerin, whey, and casein which sneak their way into a variety of food products.

So, what's the difference between vegetarian and vegan?

The definition of vegetarianism has come to mean someone who abstains from eating meat, but who still consumes milk, eggs, and other animal by-products. The term lacto-vegetarian means a vegetarian who drinks milk, while ovo-vegetarian means one who eats eggs.

No vegetarian consumes animal flesh, including broths and gravies, and some do not consume gelatin either. Many vegetarians also avoid cheese, since it's typically processed with rennet, which is derived from the stomach of calves.

One difference between veganism and vegetarianism lies in the consumption of certain animal products, though the term "strict vegetarian" usually refers to someone who eats an entirely vegan diet. Vegans don't eat milk, eggs, or honey; vegetarians often do.

However, the main difference between the two is that veganism is a lifestyle, whereas vegetarianism is a diet. Vegans don't wear animals or use them for entertainment, and seek to avoid using them in their day to day lives. With vegetarianism, one simply doesn't eat flesh and that's where it ends.

A vegan is generally dedicated to using no animal products at all. This would include avoiding wearing leather shoes, leather clothes, jackets, gloves, and consuming no animal products such as eggs, cheese, fish. They eat purely fruits and vegetables, nuts, seeds, grains, and beans.

Modern culture has perpetuated a protein myth, propagating the idea that we need large amounts of protein on a daily basis, yet this may, in fact, contribute to modern illness. When we simplify our diet and the body begins taking in its nutrition in a simpler way, we actually utilize simpler forms of protein, as long as we get a good variety.

A vegetarian enjoys a somewhat more complex diet. Generally, they consume all fruits and vegetables, grains, nuts, seeds, and beans. However, they may also include dairy products such as eggs, cheese, and milk.

A vegetarian who eats dairy products is called a lacto-vegetarian; one consuming eggs, milk and cheese is called lacto-ovo-vegetarian. Some may also consume fish, and they might say "I don't eat anything with legs."

Experimenting and becoming dedicated to vegan or vegetarian practices can be a dance or an art, as you choose a lifestyle that harmonizes with your spiritual, environmental, and dietary beliefs and commitments. Often, vegans and vegetarians may have a spiritual commitment not to kill in order to eat.

From a health standpoint, it is a growth process and a journey of experimenting to find what works for each person's body. Genetic heritage, blood type, and environmental habits and exposure all play a role in our adaptability to such dietary practices.

It is learning how to do this dance, how to find what works for our own bodies, for our own growth processes that helps us cultivate dietary choices and a lifestyle we can live with on a daily basis.

Popular healthful dietary practices today often include a range of various stages of transition into vegan, vegetarian, and all raw lifestyles. These dietary practices are being proven today to give us greater health, youth, and longevity.

We have so many foods available at all times of the year in our modern world that we have the luxury of enjoying diverse vegan and vegetarian foods.

CHAPTER 6

FAMOUS VEGANS

The vegan lifestyle has become increasingly popular over the last few decades, in particular with the rich and the famous. If there is a particular actor or actress you admire due to his or her flawless skin, sparkling eyes, and astounding beauty, it may very well be that this person owes his or her health and beauty to the vegan diet.

In fact, there are so many famous celebrity vegans today, that it is hard to keep track of them all, and the number just keeps on growing. Let's see who these famous vegans are, why they chose a vegan lifestyle, and what lessons you can learn from their lifestyle decisions to gain similarly remarkable health and wellbeing.

Observing their lifestyle choices can provide you with motivation and inspiration to try the vegan diet yourself.

The vegan diet comes to the forefront of society with the many vegan celebrities. They give reasons for their diet changes, such as choosing to not support animal cruelty. Another reason is their health and looks, a big issue for celebrities who are in television and movies.

Ellen DeGeneres - both Ellen DeGeneres and her spouse, Portia de Rossi, are vegans because of their love for animals. Once they saw a documentary on caged animals, after which Ellen DeGeneres said it was an easy decision for them to □uit eating meat and dairy products.

Mike Tyson - Mike Tyson has converted to a vegan diet, slimming down in the process, while also spending hours in the gym to build up his strength. His reason was a desire to remove "drama" from his life and become a better person through the benefits of a vegan diet.

Demi Moore - anyone who knows Demi Moore should not be surprised that she is a vegan. What is a surprise is the fact she is one celebrity who is now part of the new raw vegan food movement that is entering mainstream America.

Alicia Silverstone - Alicia has been quoted as saying "Going vegan is the single best thing I've done in my life. I am so much happier and more confident. I made a decision based on my moral beliefs."

Sandra Oh - one of the top doctors on Grey's Anatomy, Sandra Oh is also a vegan and has promoted this diet with her co-stars by taking them out to a 100% cruelty free lunch at the "True Vegan" in Hollywood. She feels that it is a lifestyle, not a dietary choice.

Woody Harrelson - when Woody Harrelson went on his vegan diet, he saw an increase in energy and a new healthy glow to his skin. His diet included raw beans, nuts, and vegetables. When he was a teenager, he had terrible skin problems and gave up dairy products at the suggestion of a friend. From that time on, his health and skin improved.

Joaquin Phoenix – this is the vegan actor who played Johnny Cash in "Walking the Line". His sister Summer is married to Casey Affleck (Ben's younger brother), who is also vegan and is planning on opening a vegan restaurant in L.A.

KD Lang - the famous singer KD Lang was subjected to violent bomb threats and burning pictures of her on her mother's lawn when she went on a meat free diet. "Who would have thought people who slaughter cattle with their bare hands could be violent?"

Tobey Maguire - Tobey has been meat free since 1992. When he had to bulk up for his role in Spiderman, he got his protein by eating lots of tofu.

All of these famous celebrity vegans became vegan for a variety of reasons, ranging from health and beauty, animal rights, and fitness. These celebrities are all aware of the many benefits of the vegan diet, and are willing to maintain this healthy lifestyle for obvious reasons.

Some of the most well-reported benefits and positive side-effects of the vegan lifestyle are weight loss, increased energy, increased focus and concentration, flawless acne-free skin, anti-aging qualities, and a reduction in allergies.

The benefits of the vegan diet are obvious, and whether the motivation is health and beauty, weight loss, increased fitness and energy, an ability to concentrate better, or animal rights, you can be sure that the vegan diet will the ideal lifestyle choice.

Famous vegans like those mentioned in this chapter can provide us with an immense amount of motivation and inspiration to make the switch to the vegan diet. The healthy bodies, clear skin, and healthy lifestyles of these celebrities are a perfect reflection of what they are eating.

CHAPTER 7

VEGAN RECIPES

With veganism becoming increasingly popular in this day and age, many folks on the vegan diet are in desperate need of quick and easy vegan recipes to accommodate their busy lifestyle.

Fortunately, over the past couple of decades, an abundance of vegan recipe ideas and information has emerged to cater to the needs of this ever-growing population of vegans. Below are some ☐uick and easy vegan recipe ideas for your breakfasts, lunches, and dinners.

1. Pancakes

Stir together in a bowl: 1 cup flour, 1 tbsp. sugar, 2 tbsp. baking powder, and a pinch of salt. Add 1 cup soy/rice/coconut milk and 2 tbsp. oil. Mix ingredients until batter is smooth. In a hot, oiled frying pan, pour in large spoonfuls of the mixture.

Flip pancakes when bubbles start to appear (approximately 2 minutes per side). Add more oil to frying pan as needed. Serve pancakes with maple syrup, agave nectar, molasses, soy yogurt, fruit, berries, or another topping of your choice.

2. Fruit smoothie

For those who have a blender, making a breakfast smoothie is a super easy and quick vegan breakfast option.

Simply blend together your choice of a mixture of the following ingredients: soy/rice/coconut milk, soy/coconut yogurt, berries, bananas, dates, raisins, maple syrup, molasses, agave nectar, cocoa powder, grated vegan chocolate, flaked/slivered almonds, crushed brazil nuts, flax seeds, LSA mix, oats, ice cubes. Serve in a tall glass.

3. Tofu & vegetable stir-fry

Cook tofu-nuggets in a hot oiled pan over high heat for 3 minutes or until golden and cooked through. Remove from pan. Next, stir fry (in peanut oil for taste) some sliced carrots, baby-corn, snow-peas, broccoli or other vegetables of choice on high heat for approximately 1 minute.

Next, add a few large tbsps. (up to ¼ cup) of vegetable stock to pan, as you continue to toss the vegetables and cook for 3-4 minutes. Add tofu back into pan and continue to stir-fry for 1 minute more. Add salt and pepper plus 1-2 tsp. sesame oil to taste. Eat by itself or with rice or noodles.

4 The grandiose garden salad

If you are sick of salads, maybe you should start to gourmet them up a little more. Nobody can get tired of eating a proper sustaining and mighty flavorsome salad.

To make the grandiose garden salad, add the following ingredients to a large bowl: 1 large packet of spinach and arugula leaves, and chopped vine-ripened tomatoes or cherry tomatoes.

Add a few spoonfuls of finely chopped sun-dried tomatoes, pitted olives, 1-2 chopped avocados, 1 finely sliced large cucumber, 1 cob of corn (either cooked or raw - kernels removed before adding to salad), ½ very thinly sliced red onion, julienned baby beetroot, and ½ cup of walnuts.

To make the dressing, combine 2 tbsp. olive oil, 1-2 tsp. lemon juice or balsamic vinegar, salt and pepper. Gently stir dressing into the salad. Enjoy the salad by itself or with some toasted sourdough bread.

5. Veggie burger/lentil burger

A veggie or lentil burger is a healthy, easy and super delicious vegan lunch idea. Find a brand of vegan patties that you like and cook the patties in a frying pan or in the oven according to packet directions.

In the meantime, slice open your bread roll and add either pesto, hummus, or guacamole to the bottom half. Add your cooked patty and top with sliced tomato, grated beetroot and carrot, and sliced pineapple. And voila, that's it!

6. Vegan Mediterranean pizza

This is a super easy vegan lunch to prepare. You can make it the night before or the day of if you are at home. Purchase a vegan pizza crust and vegan tomato paste from your local health shop. Brush your pizza crust with the tomato paste (or simply olive oil or pesto if you don't have vegan tomato paste).

Add some olives, sun-dried tomatoes, cherry tomatoes (halved), sliced mushrooms, thinly sliced red onion, and a few dollops of pesto. Next, you can either grate some vegan cheese on top or make a 'white sauce.' To make your white sauce, add 1 tbsp. flour and 1 tbsp. olive oil to a hot frying pan, and cook the mixture for about 30 seconds. Next, add some sea salt, pepper, and dried herbs, and finally, add rice or soy milk slowly to the mixture a little bit at a time, stirring consistently. When it reaches the desired thickness, take your sauce off the heat and spoon it onto your pizza. Cook your pizza in a moderately hot oven for about 30 minutes.

7. Pita bread with falafel and hummus dip

Purchase some pita bread wraps, and some falafel mixture from the supermarket or from the health shop. Prepare and fry your falafel patties as per packet directions, take them off the heat, and set aside. Spread some vegan hummus dip (from the supermarket, or make your own) on both inside surfaces of your pita bread.

Add sliced onion, shredded lettuce, parsley, grated carrot, or whatever salad ingredients you like. Put 2 or 3 falafel patties inside your pita bread, and gently break them apart with a fork. Add salt and pepper.

8. Faux lunch-meat or 'bacon' sandwich with salad

Vegan fake meat brands from the supermarkets and health shops have improved drastically in taste and ingredients over the last few years. What used to taste bland and unappetizing now has the potential to taste gourmet and enjoyable.

Faux meats, sausages, and lunch-meats now boast robust flavors (i.e. not just soy, wheat, and pea protein!), including special grains (quinoa, kamut), lentils, chickpeas, beans and herbs and spices.

Choose your favorite faux meat or cook your faux bacon. Choose your vegan bread roll, wrap, or bread and add your choice of the following gourmet ingredients: olives, sun-dried tomatoes, mustard, hummus, pesto, avocado, guacamole, lettuce or spinach, grated carrot, beetroot, corn, sliced onion, vegan cheese, fresh or dried herbs, and, of course, freshly ground pepper and sea salt.

9. Terrific tofu stir fry

Tofu is a great source of soy protein, and you can use it in almost every recipe that calls for meat or eggs. You can make a delicious lunch or dinner meal by cubing firm tofu, frying it in vegetable oil and raw soy sauce, and adding all the organic veggies of your choice: carrots, eggplant, zucchini, cabbage, bean sprouts, pea pods, and onions.

Serve over organically grown rice or brown rice, and you have a super healthy, hearty meal to fill up even the hungriest appetite.

10. Cool cold cereals

Try a bowl of Cheerios, 1 cup soy milk, and a handful of fresh strawberries or raspberries. Craving something sweeter? Cocoa beans are organic, so why not have a bowl of Cocoa Puffs or

Cocoa Krispies with 1 cup vanilla soy milk. Ultimately, you can use any of your favorite cold cereals and fruit here, so use your imagination and go nuts!

11. Awesome acai smoothie

How about an awesome fruit smoothie for lunch or for a snack? If you can find them, acai berries are native to Brazil, and it is one of the super healthy foods we don't find often around here. You can also use blueberries if acai is not available.

Blend them, fresh or frozen, with any other fruit you want (pineapples, mangoes, bananas, strawberries, etc). Add some ice or soy sorbet and blend some more. Top it with some granola and fruit slices for a super cool energy boost.

12. Cosmic curried kale

Everyone should get more greens in their diet anyway, right? Destem and wash curly kale, put it in a bowl with a shredded carrot, and then blend it with 1 part Nama Shoyu (raw soy sauce), 1 part lemon juice, 1 part olive oil, 2 cloves garlic, and cumin and coriander to taste for the dressing. Super simple and totally organic.

13. Cookoo for cocoa pudding

We all love chocolate, and the classic chocolate pudding is no exception. Even vegans can enjoy this well-known dessert. Mix 2 cups soy milk with 3 tablespoons organic cocoa, 5 tablespoons cornstarch, 1/2 cup sugar, and 1 teaspoon vanilla until smooth.

Cook it over medium heat until it thickens. Pour it into serving dishes and chill in the fridge! Now that's super easy and should satisfy any chocolate lover's cravings!

14. Roasted asparagus soup

Preheat oven to 425 degrees F. Trim and cut 2½ lbs. of thin asparagus, and cut it into 2" pieces. In a heavy roasting pan combine the asparagus with the white and light green parts of 2 leaks (cleaned and finely chopped), 2 tbsp. olive oil, and salt and pepper to taste. Mix to combine.

Bake, stirring occasionally, for 30 to 35 minutes or until leeks are golden brown and asparagus are tender.

Transfer the vegetables to a blender and 2½ cup vegetable broth. Process until completely pureed, taste to adjust seasonings.

Pour soup into shot glasses & garnish with chives if desired.

15. Waldorf salad

Peel and core 3-4 Granny Smith apples and cut into thin strips, reserving a few slices of apple with the skin on for decoration. Toss the apple slices in lemon juice to prevent apples from turning brown.

Combine 2 stalks of celery (chopped), apple slices, 4 oz. chopped walnuts or pecans, and mixed greens and toss with French vinaigrette dressing.

16. French vinaigrette dressing

Combine 2 tbsp. Dijon mustard, 2 tbsp. champagne vinegar, 6 tbs. extra-virgin olive oil, and salt and fresh ground pepper to taste in a cruet. Mix well and serve with salad.

17. Vegan blueberry pancake with veggie sausage

Pour 1 tbsp. olive oil into a non-stick, deep and large skillet. Add 1 lb. of veggie sausage and cook over medium heat until brown. Remove from heat, place in a strainer to drain, and set aside.

In a large mixing bowl, sift together 3 cups flour, 3 level tsp. baking powder, 2 tbsp. sugar, and ½ tsp. salt. Add 5 tbsp. oil and whisk in soy milk until desired thickness and consistency. Add 1½ cup mashed blueberries and mix well.

Pour ¼ cupfuls of batter into a greased skillet placed over medium heat and cook for about 3 minutes on each side till golden brown.

Place on a platter and serve hot with a veggie sausage on the side. The recipe makes 5 to 6 servings, so there is enough for everyone, or you can just enjoy breakfast in bed with that extra special someone.

18. Bell pepper soup

Combine 1½ cup sliced and seeded green or red bell pepper, 4 cloves chopped garlic, 1 large sliced onion, ¾ cup tomato paste, and 3 cups vegetable stock in a large pot and bring to a boil while stirring constantly. Reduce heat and simmer until bell peppers have softened. Drain or strain the mixture and set aside the li☐uid.

Puree the leftover bits and combine the puree with the liquid and 2 tbsp. chopped basil in a large saucepan or pot and garnish with chopped green part of spring onion. Sprinkle salt and pepper to taste. Serve hot.

19. Green smoothies

Next to water, green smoothies are one of the best things for quenching thirst. They can be easily prepared with combinations of fresh fruits and vegetables. When fresh, they are sweet enough to make adding sugar unnecessary. They are now a popular health trend, as they are good for the immune system, for detoxifying, for cleansing and energizing the body, and for weight loss.

Coconut water can be blended with spinach, and mango. You can experiment with combinations of other fruits and greens to discover your favorite flavors. This is so easy to do with modern blenders and other kitchen gadgets.

20. Vegan hummus:

This renowned Middle Eastern dip, can be a great appetizer or snack. To make hummus, you need 5 cups cooked garbanzo beans, 2 garlic cloves, 2 green onions, olive oil, lemon juice, cumin, salt and pepper, roasted sesame tahini, paprika, and pine nuts for garnish.

Prepare the hummus by processing the garbonzo beans with other ingredients in a blender. Transfer the blended paste into a bowl and drizzle with a little olive oil. Sprinkle a little paprika and pine nuts over the prepared hummus for flavor.

If you want your hummus spicier, you can add sliced red chili. Enjoy with warm, soft pitas.

21. Mushroom barley soup:

Heat 4 tsp. oil in a large pot. Add 2 cups chopped onion, 2 cloves garlic, 2 tsp. coriander, 2 carrots, and 600 g mushrooms to the pot and cook over medium heat. When vegetables are tender, add dried herbs, 1 cup barley, and 4 cups vegetable broth. Bring everything to a boil and simmer for 20 minutes until barley is soft.

22. Vegan pizza: Grab a couple of pre-made pizza crusts from the store or make your own in the kitchen. Cover in plain tomato sauce and fake cheese and cut into very thin strips. This makes a great savory snack for children.

23. Blueberry pancakes. To make this dish, simply combine two cups unbleached white flour, three tablespoons sugar, three tablespoons baking powder, and one teaspoon salt in a large bowl.

Add 2 cups vanilla soy milk and 3 tbsp. canola oil to the dry mixture and stir it all together until the batter is smooth. On the side, prepare a bowl full of 1/2 cup frozen or fresh blueberries. Ladle the batter onto a hot pancake griddle or skillet, immediately adding blueberries on top. Cook 2-3 minutes per side and serve warm.

24. Potatoes and bacon. To make a potato and "bacon" hash, dice 4 medium white potatoes, place them into a pot, cover them with water, and bring them to boil over medium heat. Allow them to boil for 10 to 15 minutes, then drain and rinse them with cold water.

While the potatoes cool, heat 1 tablespoon of olive oil over medium heat in a small skillet. Add 8 ounces of tempeh that has been cut into 1/2 inch cubes, along with 1½ tablespoons soy sauce and 1½ tablespoons liquid smoke.

Cook the mixture until all liquid has been absorbed, then flip the pieces of tempeh over and sprinkle with the remaining soy sauce and liquid smoke.

Cook until the tempeh is crispy. Finally, heat 3 tbsp. olive oil in a large skillet, adding one diced onion and the potatoes to the hot oil. Cook approximately 10 minutes before stirring in the tempeh, salt and pepper. Serve hot

25. Vegan crock pot chili

In slowcooker, combine 1 -2 cups chopped onion, 1 medium chopped green bell pepper, 1 can each pinto beans and kidney beans with liquid, 1 can dices tomatoes, 1-2 tbsp. spicy chili pepper, 1 diced jalapeno, and salt and pepper to taste. Mix well and cook on high for 4-5 hours or on low for 6-8 hours.

26. Vegan slow cooker lasagna

Slice 1 large yellow squash and 1 large zucchini into thin lengthwise strips using a mandolin. Layer the vegetable "noodles," in the crock pot with vegan ricotta (see below), 3-4 cups organic tomato basil sauce and 1-2 cups vegan pizza-style shredded cheese. Continue layering until all the ingredients are gone, making sure the last two layers are sauce and cheese. Cook on high for 4-5 hours or 6-8 on low.

Make the vegan ricotta by blending 14 oz. extra firm tofu with lemon juice, sugar, basil, salt and garlic powder to taste

CONCLUSION

Becoming vegan is an expression of profound reverence for life. It is a gradual process that takes oplace as we learn about the many sources of animal products in our lives. Becoming vegan is a transformational act, a both life-changing and life-affirming decision.

Practicing a vegan lifestyle is the single most important thing we can do for animals, as well as for our health, and it is something that each of us has the power to do. It is also a wonderful way to start the new year, and not only is it a healthy decision for you, but it's also a healthy decision for the environment.

Veganism denotes a philosophy and a way of life that seeks to exclude, as far as is possible and practical, all forms of exploitation of and cruelty to animals for food, clothing, or any other purpose.

Veganism works to expose and end the subtle indoctrination of industries that wish to desensitize humanity to the violence against the many for the gain of the few.

Vegans withhold economic and moral support from any enterprise that involves the abuse or exploitation of animals (such as zoos or circuses) or humans (such as sweatshops). Vegans also reject the use of living creatures as instruments or materials for teaching, scientific inquiry, entertainment, or other utilitarian purposes.

Vegan clothing, shoes, outerwear, and accessories are either plant-based or synthetic, and vegans do not wear or use leather or the skins, fur, feathers, shells, or secretions of any creatures.

Vegan foods, such as whole grains, vegetables, fruits, and beans, are low in fat, contain no cholesterol, and are rich in fiber and nutrients. Vegans do not consume eggs or dairy products, and they avoid animal ingredients in clothing and other consumer goods.

Vegans cannot live by bean sprouts alone: Most new vegetarians and vegans significantly increase the amount and variety of fresh fruits and vegetables in their diet.

Vegan milks are rapidly growing in popularity and can be found in nearly all supermarkets. Among vegan milks, soymilk and rice milk are most common, but there are also vegan milks made from almonds or oats, and more varieties are sure to come.

Vegan cookies, donuts, candy bars, and Pop Tart-type treats are readily available. Vegans eat about 40-50 grams of fiber per day (on average).

Veganism holds that the simple fact that animals can't speak English (or Spanish or Chinese or Russian) is not a valid reason to exploit them. Becoming vegan is the embodiment of meaningful activism.

Veganism, the natural extension of vegetarianism, is an integral component of a cruelty-free lifestyle, and emerges as the lifestyle most consistent with the philosophy that animals are not ours to exploit.

Becoming vegan is one of the most environmentally responsible choices you will ever make, as well as one of the best and healthiest things you can do for your body.

Becoming vegan is actually very easy, and while you might think you'll miss the meat, I assure you, after a few weeks, you really won't.

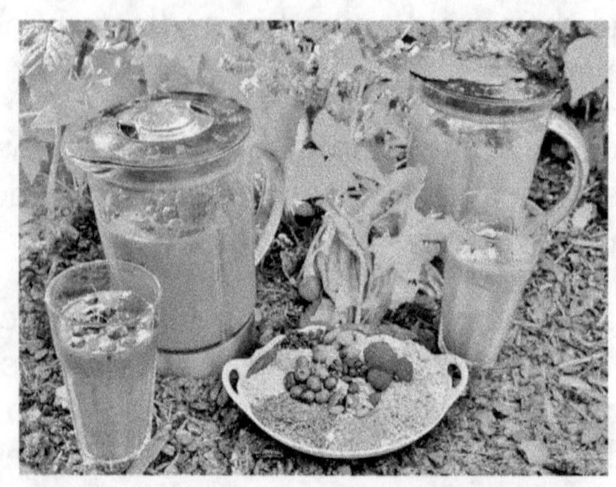

Thanks for reading!